Paleo

The Magic Ways To Lose Weight And Eat Healthy Food,
Including Step By Step Guides To Meal Plans

(Paleo Recipes For Beginners To Lose Weight And Get
Healthy Lifestyle)

Darin Hogan

TABLE OF CONTENTS

Spice Infused Mashed Potatoes

Ingredients:

2 Little Large sized Potatoes

1/2 tsp green Chili paste

1/2 tsp Clove powder

1/2 tsp Cinnamon powder

1/2 tsp Cumin seed powder

2 cup Curd

2 tsp Honey

Salt to taste

2 tbsp fresh Coriander leaves

Instructions:

Cook the potatoes in boiling water.

Once they are boiled, remove the skin and mash the potatoes to a thick paste.

Add the chili paste, clove powder, cinnamon powder, cumin seed powder, curd and honey to the mashed potatoes.

Add salt and mix well, garnish with fresh coriander leaves before serving.

Potatoes In Green Fresh Lemon Chutney

Ingredients:

1/2 tsp Cumin seeds

1/2 tsp Asafetida

2 tsp grated coconut pulp

2-4 tbsp Cooking Oil

2 Little Large sized Potatoes

1/2 tsp green Chili paste

4 tbsp fresh Coriander leaves

2 tsp fresh Fresh lemon juice

1/2 tsp Coriander seed powder

Salt to taste

Instructions:

1. Make holes in the potatoes with a fork and then boil them in water.
2. Once the potatoes are cooked, peel off the skin and cut them into small bite size pieces.

3. Making *Green Fresh lemon Chutney* –

4. Grind chili paste and coriander leaves into a thick paste. Add fresh lemon juice and coriander seed powder to the paste. This is the green fresh lemon chutney.
5. Mix the green fresh lemon chutney, salt and potatoes in a bowl and stir well.
6. Heat the cooking oil in a pan.
7. Once the oil is hot, add the cumin seeds and asafetida.
8. When cumin starts to crackle, turn off the heat and add the contents of the pan to the chutney coated potatoes in the bowl.

9. Mix well and garnish with grated coconut pulp.

Green Potato Kebab

Ingredients:

2 cup fresh Coriander leaves (finely chopped)

2 tsp Ginger-Garlic paste

1/2 tsp Coriander seed powder

Salt to taste

5-10 tbsp Cooking Oil

2-4 Little Large sized Potatoes

2 cups fresh Green Peas

1 tsp green Chilly paste

2 cups fresh Spinach leaves

2 cup Cottage Cheese (finely grated)

Instructions:

1. Boil the Potatoes and green peas.

2. Remove the skin of the potatoes and mash them into a thick paste.

3. Also mash the peas into a paste and mix it thoroughly with the mashed potatoes.

4. Finely chop the spinach leaves, mix them with grated cottage cheese.

5. Once thoroughly mixed add the chili paste, chopped coriander leaves, coriander seed powder and ginger-garlic paste.

6. Then add this green kebab mixture to the potato-green pea paste.

7. Once mixed thoroughly make small balls of this mixture.

8. (keep the size of the balls small so that they will be thoroughly cooked when shallow fried)

9. Heat the cooking oil in a pan.

10. Once the oil is hot, put the green kebab balls into the pan and shallow fry them, serve hot.

Crispy Sour Plantains

Ingredients:

2 plantains

2 tbsp Tamarind pulp

4 -4 tbsp Cooking Oil

Salt to taste

1/2 tsp red Chili powder

2 cup Rice flour

Instructions:

1. Remove the skin of the plantains and slice them into thin wheels.
2. Rub salt, red chili powder and tamarind pulp to these slices thoroughly and leave the slices to marinate for 45-50 min.
3. Heat the cooking oil in a pan.

4. Once the oil is hot, shallow fry the slices (dip the slices in dry rice flour, before shallow frying)
5. Fry till crispy. Garnish with fresh coriander leaves and serve hot.

Carrot Chutney

Ingredients:

230 gm fresh Carrots

4 tbsp Sesame seeds

1/2 tsp Asafetida

1/2 tsp Mustard seeds

1/2 tsp Turmeric powder

1/2 tsp Cumin seeds

1/2 tsp red Chili powder

1 cup of grated Coconut pulp (dried)

4 tbsp roughly grated Almonds

2-4 Curry leaves

1/2 tsp Sugar

2-4 tbsp Cooking Oil

Instructions:

1. Finely grate the carrots, then spread them over a flat tray and sun-dry them for a few hours till the moisture dries up.
2. Heat the cooking oil in a pan.
3. Once the oil is hot, add the cumin seeds, asafetida, mustard seeds and turmeric powder.
4. Once the cumin starts crackling, add the curry leaves followed by the dried grated carrots, sesame seeds and grated almonds.

5. Stir for a minute and then add grated coconut pulp, red chili powder, sugar and salt.
6. Don't cover the pan and stir the carrots till they become crispy.

Crunchy-Sour Cucumber

Ingredients:

2 tbsp grated Coconut pulp

2 tbsp fresh Coriander leaves

2-4 tsp fresh fresh lemon juice

1/2 tsp Sugar

1/2 tsp Cumin seeds

2-4 tbsp Cooking Oil

250 gm fresh Cucumbers

4 tbsp roughly grated Almonds

11

1/2 tsp green Chili powder

Salt to taste

Instructions:

1. Peel off the skin of the cucumbers and finely slice them into thin slices.
2. Put these slices in a bowl.
3. Heat the cooking oil in a pan.
4. Once the oil is hot, add the cumin seeds and green chili paste, stir for a minute and then pour the contents of the pan over the cucumber slices.
5. Then add grated coconut pulp, chopped coriander leaves, sugar and salt to the cucumber slices and stir well.
6. Then add the fresh lemon juice to the cucumber, stir a bit and serve fresh.

Instant Cucumber Pickle

Ingredients:

1/2 tsp Asafetida

1/2 tsp Turmeric powder

1/2 tsp red Chili powder

2 tbsp Coriander leaves (finely chopped)

2 tsp Salt

2-4 tbsp Cooking Oil

230 gm fresh Cucumber

2 tsp Mustard seeds

1 tsp Fenugreek seeds

2-4 tsp Fresh lemon juice

Instructions:

1. Peel off the skin of the cucumbers and finely dice them in small bite sized pieces.
2. Remove them in a bowl.
3. Then sprinkle turmeric powder, red chili powder and salt over the cucumbers and leave it for 8-25 minutes.
4. You will notice that cucumber secrets fair amount of water.
5. Remove this water in a cup.
6. Do not throw this water away. Grind 1 tsp of fenugreek seeds and 1 tsp of mustard seed in this water into a paste.
7. Rub this paste evenly to the diced cucumbers and also add the fresh lemon juice to the diced cucumbers.
8. Heat the cooking oil in a pan.
9. Once the oil is hot, add the remaining mustard seeds and asafetida to the pan and stir for a minute.

10. When mustard seeds crackle, add the contents of the pan to the cucumbers and mix well.
11. Garnish with coriander leaves and serve fresh.

Coconut-Bengal Gram Chutney

Ingredients:

1 cup fresh Curd

1/2 tsp Mustard seeds

1/2 tsp Asafetida

2-4 tbsp Cooking Oil

2 Curry leaves

Salt to taste

2 cup fresh grated Coconut pulp

2 tbsp split Bengal Grams

2 tbsp split Black Grams

1 tsp green Chili paste

Instructions:

1. Soak bengal grams and black grams for at least 2 hrs, then keep them on a strainer to let all water drain off.
2. Heat the cooking oil in a pan.
3. Once the oil is hot, add the mustard seeds, curry leaves and asafetida to the pan.
4. When the mustard seeds start to crackle add the bengal gram and black gram to the pan, stir it for a while and then cover the pan with a lid and let it cook for 8 -8 minutes.
5. Once it is cooked, remove the lid and add the green chili paste, stir for a few seconds and then put the lid back on and cook for minute or so.
6. Then remove the lid and add the grated coconut pulp to the pan and mix it all well, stir for a minute more and then turn-off the heat.

7. Once it cools down, add the curd and salt to it, mix thoroughly and serve with a garnish of chopped fresh coriander leaves.

Green Mango Chutney

Ingredients:

4 tbsp fresh Coriander leaves (finely chopped)

1 tbsp Olive Oil

Salt to taste

2 Little Large sized raw green mangoes

4 tbsp grated Coconut pulp

1/2 tsp green Chili paste

Instructions:

Finely grate the raw mangoes.

Then add the grated coconut pulp and green chili paste to the grated mangoes and mix it well.

Then add the olive oil and mix again.

Then add the salt to this mixture and mix again.

You'll notice that a lot of water is secreted by the mangoes, when you add salt. (don't remove this water)

Potato Chutney

Ingredients:

2 tbsp fresh Coriander leaves (chopped)

1/2 tsp asafetida

1/2 tsp Turmeric powder

19

2 Little Large sized Potato

1/2 tsp green Chili paste

4 tbsp grated Coconut pulp

Instructions:

1. Boil the potato for a few minutes in water. (don't cook it completely, just let it remain in boiling water for some time.)
2. Then peel off its skin and finely grate it.
3. Add green chili paste, grated coconut, chopped coriander leaves and salt to the potatoes and mix well.
4. Then add asafetida and turmeric powder to this mixture and grind it into a thick coarse paste.

Ripe Mango In Sour Sauce

Ingredients:

1/2 tsp Mustard seeds

2 tsp Tamarind Pulp

1/2 tsp Sugar

2 Little Large size Ripe Mango

1 cup fresh grated Coconut pulp

1/2 tsp red Chili powder

Salt

Instructions:

1. Remove the skin of the mango and cut it into small pieces.
2. Grind grated coconut pulp, mustard seeds, red chili powder and salt into a thick paste. (add 2-4 tsp water while grinding)

21

3. Add the mango to this paste and mix well.
4. Then add the tamarind pulp and sugar finally. Stir well till sugar dissolves.
5. Serve while fresh.

Spicy Pineapple Stew

Ingredients:

1 tsp Cumin seeds

1/2 tsp Mustard seeds

1/2 tsp Turmeric powder

2-4 tbsp Cooking Oil

4 cup ripe Pineapple (finely diced)

2 tbsp grated Jaggery

1/2 tsp red Chili powder

2 cup grated Coconut pulp

2 Curry Leaves

Salt to taste

Instructions:

1. Grind grated coconut pulp, 1/2 tsp cumin seeds, 1/2 tsp mustard seeds together into a thick paste.
2. Add 2 cup of water to a pan and bring it to a boil, then add the diced pineapple, turmeric powder, red chili powder and salt to the water and let it cook for 5-10 minutes.
3. Then add jaggery to it and stir till it dissolves and then add the paste we have made earlier and mix well. This is the stew base.
4. Heat the cooking oil in another pan.
5. Once the oil is hot, add the cumin seeds, curry leaves.
6. Once the cumin starts crackling, pour the contents of the pan to the stew

base and stir for a bit and then turn off the heat under the stew.

7. The Pineapple stew is ready, serve hot.

Stirred Cabbage With Black Gram

Ingredients:

1 tsp Asafetida

1 tsp Mustard seeds

2-4 Curry leaves

 Salt to taste

2-4 tbsp Cooking Oil

2 Little Large sized Cabbage

2 tbsp split Black Gram

2 dried red chili

Instructions:

1. Soak the split Black Gram overnight.
2. Clean the Cabbage and chop it finely into thin strips.
3. Heat the cooking oil in a pan.
4. Once the oil is hot, add Curry leaves, Mustard seeds, asafetida and the dried chili.
5. Once the Mustard seeds start crackling, add the split Black Gram.
6. Lower the flame and stir the contents in the pan for a couple of minutes.
7. Then add the chopped Cabbage to the pan, add salt to taste and cover the pan with a lid and serve hot once the cabbage is cooked.

Curd Cooked Bitter Gourd

Ingredients:

2 tsp Turmeric powder

1/2 tsp Cumin seeds

1/2 tsp Mustard seeds

1/2 tsp Asafetida

2-4 tbsp Cooking Oil

2 cups of Curd

250 gm Bitter Gourd

1/2 tsp Coriander seed powder

1/2 tsp red Chili powder

Instructions:

1. Cut and clean the bitter gourd
2. Wash it with water and then grate the bitter gourd.

3. Add turmeric and salt to the bitter gourd; mix it well and leave for 2 hr.

4. After an hour squeeze out all the water from the bitter gourd.

5. Heat the cooking oil in a pan.

6. Once the oil is hot, add the cumin seeds, mustard seeds, asafetida and chili powder.

7. After the mustard seeds start crackling add the bitter gourd to the pan.

8. Stir well and cover up with a lid and let it cook over its own steam.

9. After a few minutes add the curd and coriander seed powder to the pan

10. Keep stirring the contents of the pan continuously till the bitter gourd is completely cooked.

11. Serve while hot.

Flour Infused Snake Gourd

Ingredients:

1/2 tsp Turmeric powder

1/2 tsp Cumin seeds

1/2 tsp Mustard seeds

1/2 tsp Asafetida

2-4 tbsp Cooking Oil

270 gm fresh Snake Gourd

2 Little Large Onion

1 cup Chickpea flour

1/2 tsp Coriander seed powder

1/2 tsp red Chili powder

Instructions:

1. Peel off the skin of the snake gourd, remove the seeds and dice it finely and then clean it with water.
2. Finely dice the onion.
3. Heat the cooking oil in a pan.
4. Once the oil is hot, add the cumin seeds, mustard seeds, asafetida and chili powder.
5. Once the mustard starts crackling, add the diced fresh onion and stir till it becomes pink.
6. Add the snake gourd, stir for 2 minutes then add the coriander seed powder and Turmeric powder.
7. Add salt to taste, and place a lid on it to allow the snake gourd to cook over its own steam.
8. After a few minutes, remove the lid and sprinkle over the chickpea flour while continuously stirring.

9. Once you've added all the flour and stirred well, add 1 tbsp of cooking oil and cook till excess moisture dries up.
10. Serve while hot.

Tomato-Okra Fry

Ingredients:

230 gm fresh tender Okra's

2 Little Large Potato

2 Tomatoes

2 Green Chilly

1/2 tsp Coriander seed powder

1/2 tsp Mustard seeds

1/2 tsp Turmeric powder

1/2 tsp Asafetida

2-4 tbsp Cooking Oil

Instructions:

1. Clean the potato, peel off its skin and cut it into thin vertical strips.
2. Finely dice the tomatoes.
3. Wash the Okra and remove the hard stems, then cut it into small, thin wheels.
4. Finely chop the green chilly.
5. Heat the cooking oil in a pan.
6. Once the oil is hot, add the mustard seeds, asafetida and turmeric powder.
7. Once the mustard starts crackling, add the chopped chilly and tomatoes. Stir for a couple of minutes.
8. Then add the potato strips and stir till the potato becomes a bit red, then add the okra, coriander seed powder and salt.
9. Place a lid on the pan and let the okra cook for a few minutes.

10. Then remove the lid and stir well till all the moisture evaporates and you get a crispy okras. Serve while hot.

Stirred Radish With Green Gram

Ingredients:

1/2 tsp Coriander seed powder

1/2 tsp Mustard seeds

1/2 tsp Turmeric powder

1/2 tsp Asafetida

2-4 tbsp Cooking Oil

Salt to taste

2 fresh, tender Radishes

4 tbsp split Green Gram

2 green Chilly, finely diced

Instructions:

1. Soak the split green grams for at least 4 -4 hrs.
2. Wash the radish and finely dice it.
3. Heat the cooking oil in a pan.
4. Once the oil is hot, add the mustard seeds, asafetida and turmeric powder.
5. Once the mustard starts crackling, add the chilly followed by the soaked split green grams.
6. Stir for a couple of minutes and then add the diced radish. Sprinkle salt and coriander seed powder over the radish and stir well over a low flame.
7. Place a lid on the pan and let it cook.
8. Once the radish is cooked, remove the lid and continuously stir till the excess moisture evaporates.
9. Serve while hot.

Flour Infused Radish Leaves

Ingredients:

1/2 tsp Coriander seed powder

1/2 tsp Mustard seeds

1/2 tsp Turmeric powder

1/2 tsp Asafetida

2-4 tbsp Cooking Oil

2 bowl fresh, tender Radishes leaves

1 a cup of diced Radish

4 -4 cloves of Garlic

2 green Chilly

Salt to taste

Instructions:

1. Wash the radish leaves with water, drain the water and chop them.
2. Make a chilly-garlic paste.
3. Heat the cooking oil in a pan.
4. Once the oil is hot, add the mustard seeds, asafetida and turmeric powder.
5. Once the mustard starts crackling, add the chilly-garlic paste and stir for a minute.
6. Then add the diced radish to the pan and let it simmer for a couple of minutes.
7. Then add the radish leaves to the pan followed by the coriander seed powder and salt.
8. Place a lid over the pan and leave till the leaves are cooked.

9. Then remove the lid and stir over a low flame till the excess moisture evaporates.

10. Serve while hot.

Stirred Cucumber

Ingredients:

2-4 Curry leaves

1/2 tsp Mustard seeds

1/2 tsp Cumin seeds

1/2 tsp Asafetida

Salt to taste

2-4 tbsp Cooking Oil

4 Little Large sized Cucumbers

2 tbsp split Bengal Gram

2 green Chilly, finely chopped

1/2 tsp Coriander seed powder

Instructions:

1. Soak the split bengal grams overnight
2. De-skin the cucumbers and finely dice them.
3. Heat the cooking oil in a pan.
4. Once the oil is hot, add the cumin seeds, mustard seeds, asafetida, chilly and curry leaves.
5. Once the cumin starts crackling, add the soaked bengal gram and stir for a couple of minutes.
6. Then add the finely diced cucumbers and coriander seed powder and salt.
7. Cover the pan with a lid and let it cook over a low flame for 2 minutes.
8. Then remove the lid and keep stirring till the excess moisture dries up.
9. Serve hot.

Pumpkin With Dry Spices

Ingredients:

1/2 tsp Poppy Seeds (*Khas Khas*)

1/2 tsp Cumin seeds

1/2 tsp Asafetida

1/2 tsp Turmeric powder

Salt to taste

2-4 tbsp Cooking Oil

270 gm red Pumpkin

2 tbsp roasted Almonds, roughly grated

2 tbsp dried coconut, roughly grated

2 dried red chilly

1/2 tsp Fenugreek seeds

Instructions:

1. Peel off the skin from the pumpkin, also remove the seed and chop it into small bite size pieces.
2. Roast fenugreek seeds, poppy seeds, dried red chili and grated coconut, together in a pan for a couple of minutes. Then grind these ingredients into fine powder.
3. Heat the cooking oil in a pan.
4. Once the oil is hot, add the cumin seeds, asafetida and turmeric powder.
5. Once the cumin starts crackling, add the pumpkin to the pan followed by the dry spices powder we have created earlier.
6. Add salt to taste and cover with a lid.
7. Let it cook over steam for a few minutes, then remove the lid and keep stirring till the excess moisture dries up.
8. Serve hot.

Flour Infused Pumpkin

Ingredients:

1/2 tsp Mustard seeds

1/2 tsp Asafetida

1/2 tsp Turmeric powder

2-4 tbsp Cooking Oil

Salt to taste

230 gm red Pumpkin

2 tbsp Chickpea flour

1/2 tsp coriander seed powder

2 green chili, finely chopped

Instructions:

1. Peel off the skin from the pumpkin, also remove the seed and chop it into small bite size pieces.
2. Heat the cooking oil in a pan.
3. Once the oil is hot, add the mustard seeds, asafetida, turmeric powder and chopped chili.
4. Once the mustard starts crackling, add pumpkin, coriander seed powder and salt. Stir for a while and then put a lid on the pan and let it simmer over a low flame.
5. Once it is cooked, remove the lid and sprinkle the chickpea flour in the pan, while continuously stirring the contents of the pan.
6. Once the flour is sprinkled, add 2-4 tsp of cooking oil and then again stir till the excess moisture dries up.
7. Garnish with chopped coriander leaves and serve hot.

Stirred French Beans

Ingredients:

2-4 Curry Leaves

1/2 tsp Cumin seeds

1/2 tsp Asafetida

1/2 tsp Turmeric powder

2-4 tbsp Cooking Oil

Salt to taste

230 gm fresh French Beans

2 green chilly finely chopped

1/2 tsp Cumin seed powder

1/2 tsp Coriander seed powder

2-4 tsp Fresh Fresh lemon Juice

Instructions:

1. Clean the french beans, and chop them into small pieces.
2. Boil 1 a liter water and put the beans in it, leave for 2 minutes.
3. Remove the beans and keep them in a strainer, so the excess water drains off.
4. Heat the cooking oil in a pan.
5. Once the oil is hot, add the curry leaves, cumin seeds, asafetida, turmeric powder and chilly.
6. Once the cumin starts crackling, add the french beans followed by the coriander seed powder, Cumin seeds powder and salt.
7. Keep stirring over a low flame till all the excess water dries off, then add the fresh lemon juice, stir a few times and serve hot.

Yummy Paleo Pancake

Ingredients:

4 fresh fresh eggs, , beaten

4 mashed bananas (any variety)

2 small sized apple (peeled and diced)

4 tsp. cinnamon powder

4 tbsp. almond butter

Walnuts (optional)

1 tsp. pure vanilla extract

2 tbsp. (or more) grass-fed butter

Procedure:

1. Beat 4 fresh fresh eggs, in a bowl and add in mashed bananas.

2. Add in diced apple, walnuts and blend in the banana and egg mixture evenly.

3. Add the cinnamon powder, almond butter, and vanilla extract. Mix in the pancake batter.

4. Over Little Large heat, pre-heat a non-stick pan add melt butter, and then pour small amount of the pancake batter into the pan.

5. Cook until small bubbles appear on top, but golden brown and firm at the bottom, (for about 4 to 4 minutes). Flip and cook the other side.

6. Top with fresh fruits instead of pan cake syrup to that perfect guilt- free pancake!

Veggies And Egg Cups

Ingredients:

2 cup fresh asparagus (chopped)

2 cup spinach (chopped)

A dash of kosher salt and freshly cracked black pepper to taste

6 organic fresh eggs,

2 Little Large sized white onion

2 cup broccoli florets (chopped)

2 cup zucchini (chopped)

Procedure:

1. Preheat the oven to 4 00F. Beat fresh fresh eggs, in a mixing bowl and in a dash of salt and pepper; then stir in the chopped veggies.

2. Prepare porcelain ramekins by brushing it with oil. (*If you do not have*

51

a ramekin dish, you can use muffin pans)

3. Transfer the egg mixture into the ramekin dish and bake for 20-50 minutes or until the fresh fresh eggs are set.

4. Remove from heat and let sit for 25 minutes before serving. Top it celery.

Paleo Hamburger

Ingredients

6 fresh eggs,

4 strips of cooked bacon strips

1 lb. ground grass-fed beef

1/9 tsp. of nutmeg

1/9 tsp. of pepper

A dash of sea salt to taste

2 tsp. of fennel seeds

2 tbsp. of olive oil

Procedure:

1. In a bowl, mix together ground beef, fennel seeds, nutmeg, salt and pepper.

2. Shape it into patties and set aside.

3. Place a skillet on low to Little Large heat.

4. In the heated skillet scramble the fresh fresh eggs, shaping it into several uneven circles, flip on other side to cook. Set aside.

5. In the same pan fry beef patties until golden brown or for 4 to 6 minutes.

6. Get cooked patties from the pan.

7. Use the scrambled egg as your bread layering it with patties and bacon in between.

Homemade Paleo Corned Beef

- 2 garlic cloves (minced)
- ¾ cup beef broth
- Salt and pepper to add flavor
- 2 tbsp. olive oil
- 4 cups corned beef (cooked and chopped)
- 2 cups radishes (cut into quarters)
- 2 Little Large sized fresh onion (chopped)

Procedure:

1. Over Little Large to high fire, heat the skillet drizzled with 2 tbsp. olive oil.

2. Put in onions and sauté for 6 minutes, add in the radishes and cook for another 6 minutes.

3. Add in the garlic and continue sautéing for another minute.

4. Pour in the beef broth and then loosely cover the pan. Simmer until the radishes are tender and cooked.

5. Add in the corned beef and mix well.

6. Dash with salt and pepper to taste.

-

-

Paleo Breakfast Bake

Ingredients

2   large-sized sweet potatoes, cut 2 ” cubes

2 small tomato, sliced

4 fresh fresh eggs, (beaten)

Kosher salt and black pepper to taste

4 tbsp. bacon fat

2 lb. steak, cut into bite sized pieces

2 green bell pepper, small-sized chopped

2 small red bell pepper, chopped

Procedure:

1. Set oven to 4 8 0F
2. Heat up the bacon fat in a pan over Little Large to high heat.
3. Add in steak and cook until it turns brown. Set aside.
4. In the same pan sauté the green and red bell peppers and onions for 2 to 4 minutes.
5. Put in sweet potatoes and sautéing in all together until tender for 8 to 25 minutes.
6. Put the steak in a baking pan and stir everything together.
7. Using the back of a spoon make a small indention to the mixtures.
8. Pour the beaten fresh fresh eggs, into the indentations.

9. Add in tomatoes on top of the fresh eggs, .
10. Add salt and pepper to give a flavorful taste.
11. Put the skillet in the oven and bake for 25 minutes, or until done.

-

-

Healthy Cucumber Sandwich

Ingredients

2 Little Large sized cucumber

Dijon mustard

Spreadable garlic and herbs

4 slices of turkey breast

6 slices of crunchy bacon

1. Cut the cucumber into half and scooping out all the seeds.

2. Evenly spread the garlic and herb on the cucumber

3. Meanwhile, cook the turkey slices in a pan with 1/2 cup of water. Season with a dash of kosher salt.

4. Remove from the heat when the turkey slices are done and let it cool down for a bit.

5. Arrange the turkey slices on top of the hollow cucumber add mustard and crunchy bacon bites.

6. Place the other half on top to make a sandwich.

Tuna And Cabbage Medley

Ingredients for tuna:

2 tsp. freshly ground pepper

1 cup cassava flour

1/2 tsp. mustard powder

Sea salt to give flavor

6-8 pieces tuna fillets

4 tbsp. olive oil

2 small beaten egg

Ingredients for sautéed cabbage:

2 cups cauliflower florets

6 cloves of garlic (chopped)

2 head cabbage, sliced

63

2 tbsp. olive oil

1 cup chicken broth

Procedure:

1. Tuna Preparation:
2. Mix cassava flour, freshly ground pepper, salt and powdered mustard in a small bowl and transfer it to an empty plate.
3. Dip tuna fillets one at a time in egg and dredge with flour mixture.
4. Fry for about 2 to 4 minutes on each or until golden brown.
5. Set aside.

Cabbage Preparation:

1. Place a small pan over a low to Little Large fire. Add in oil and heat.
2. Throw in the in chopped garlic and sauté for 2 minutes.
3. Add cauliflower florets and sauté for another 4 minutes.
4. Add in cabbage and continue sautéing. Do not over cook
5. Pour over chicken stock, simmering it for 2 more minute.
6. Serve the sautéed cabbage as your side dish for healthy tuna meal.

Spicy Chicken Guacamole And Mango Salad

2 head of romaine lettuce (chopped)

2 tsp. of chili powder

1 tsp. of cumin

Salt and pepper to taste

2 to 4 cups of shredded chicken breast

2 Little Large sized mango, peeled and diced

2 Little Large sized guacamole, diced

Procedure:

1. Place the romaine lettuce into a small bowl.
2. In a separate bowl, put the shredded chicken and add a 6 tbsp. of water.
3. Cook for 30 to 25 seconds in a microwave oven over a medium-high heat.
4. After cooking, mix in the cumin and chili powder.
5. Put the chicken with cumin and chili powder into the small bowl of lettuce.
6. Top it with guacamole and mango.
7. Enjoy your meal. No need to add a dressing it is appetizing as it is.

Calvolfiore Riso

4 tbsp. bacon fat

1 cup chopped fresh cilantro

2 Little Large sized white onion, chopped (about 2 cup)

1 tsp. kosher salt

2 heads of cauliflower

1/9 tsp. ground black pepper

4 cloves garlic (chopped)

1. Chop the cauliflowers.

2. Toss into the food processor or a blender until the cauliflower pieces are the shape and size of rice.

3. Be careful not to over blend.

4. Do them by batches. When you're done set aside the chopped cauliflower.

5. Heat a medium-sized skillet over low to Little Large fire.

6. Sauté the garlic and fresh onion in oil for 2 minute.

7. Add in the chopped cauliflower mixing it well.

8. Then add the salt and pepper to flavor, sauté it for 6 more minutes or until the cauliflower is slightly tender.

9. Serve in a bowl and add some freshly chopped cilantro!

Fruity Pork Chops

6 cloves of garlic (minced)

coarse black pepper and sea salt to taste

1 tsp. garlic powder

1 tsp. fresh onion powder for flavor

4 tbsp. ghee

6 bone in pork chops

4 whole apples (Little Large sliced)

1 cup pork bone broth (you may also use chicken of beef broth)

fresh parsley (chopped)

Procedure:

1. Heat a small sized frying pan over Little Large fire. Throw in the garlic, parsley and broth and let it simmer for 2 minutes.
2. Flavor the pork chops with fresh onion powder, garlic powder, salt and black pepper.
3. Place the chops in a skillet and cook for 4 to 6 minutes or until brown spooning some of the garlic broth over the meat. Flip over and continue to cook until done.
4. In a separate frying pan, melt the ghee and sauté apples over a low to Little Large heat until it is tender.
5. Transfer the cooked apples into the other pan with pork chops and marinate together for 6 minutes to blend in the flavors.

6. Serve on a platter spooning over the pork chop broth with the apples on top.

-

Salmon In Coconut Cream Sauce

2 small diced shallot

4 gloves minced garlic

1/2 tsp. kosher salt

2 Little Large fresh lemon zest

1 cup fresh lemon juice

4 tbsp. freshly chopped basil

4 pounds salmon fillet

¾ cup full fat coconut milk

4 tbsp. coconut toil

1/2 freshly ground pepper

1. Preheat oven to 4 6 0F.

2. Place salmon fillet in a baking dish, sprinkle it with salt and freshly ground pepper on both sides.

3. Heat a pan over Little Large fire. Add the coconut oil, garlic and shallots. Cook for few more minutes until the shallots have softened.

4. Add in coconut milk, fresh lemon juice and fresh lemon zest and bring to a low boil.

5. Add in basil and reduce the heat.

6. Pour the coconut milk mixture over the salmon, baking it uncovered for about 25 to 25 minutes or until done.

7. Enjoy your healthy salmon meal!

The Caveman's Pizza

6 medium-sized mushroom, (sliced)

2 sausage cut into thick slices

25 strips of bacon cooked and crushed

2 small green bell pepper (diced)

2 cup tomato sauce, marinara sauce with no salt added

1 tsp. oregano

2 cup cherry tomatoes sliced in half

 4 cups of almond flour

4 tbsp. almond butter

4 small – sized egg (beaten)

1 tsp. kosher salt

4 tsp. olive oil

2 large- sized white fresh onion (diced)

1. Preheat the oven to 4 6 0F.

2. In a small bowl mix almond flour, egg, butter, salt and combine well.

3. Brush a baking sheet with half of the olive oil, and pour the mixture over it, and make a 1/2 thin crust and cook in the oven for 25 minutes.

4. While waiting for the crust, heat a small skillet over a Little Large fire. Add olive oil, white onions, sausages, and mushrooms and cook until brown. Remove from pan and set aside.

5. In the same pan, throw in the garlic and green pepper and sauté for a few minutes or until tender. Do not overcook.

6. Take out the crust from the oven and generously spread the marinara sauce on it. Top with sausage and sautéed veggies.

7. Sprinkle with oregano, and place in the oven for 30 to 45 minutes.

8. Remove from the oven when cooked.

9. Top with sliced tomatoes and crushed bacon.

Raspberry And Almond Muffin Cups

4 small fresh fresh eggs, (beaten)

2 cups almond butter

1 cup raw honey

1 cup silvered almonds

1 coconut oil

2 cups raspberries

1 tsp. salt

2 cups almond flour

2 tsp. baking powder

2 tsp. baking soda

2 tsp. almond extract

Procedure:

1. Preheat your oven to 4 6 0 F.
2. In a small bowl combine all of the dry ingredients together. Set aside.
3. In another bowl combine almond butter, egg, almonds, honey, almond extract, and coconut oil.
4. Gradually mix in with the dry ingredients.
5. Mix the fresh raspberries.
6. Slightly grease muffin pan with coconut oil, or line it with paper muffin liners then scoop batter evenly into 8-25 muffins cups.
7. Bake for 35 -25 minutes. Watch muffins to be sure they do not overcook.

A Perfect Fresh Fruit Salad

2 lb. black grapes (cut into halves)

2 lb. green grapes (cut into halves)

1 cup walnut and almonds (chopped)

1 tsp. cinnamon powder

2 Little Large sized oranges (peeled and diced)

2 Little Large sized apple (diced)

2 Little Large sized peach (chopped)

1. Combine all fruits in a bowl.

2. Sprinkle with chopped nuts and cinnamon.

The Paleo Banana Carrot Muffin

2 cups pitted dates

6 Little Large sized bananas

6 small fresh eggs,

2 tsp. apple cider vinegar

1 cup coconut oil

2 small carrots (grated)

2 cup walnut (finely chopped)

4 cups almond flour

4 tsp. baking soda

2 salt

2 tsp. cinnamon powder

1. Pre heat oven to 4 6 0F

2. In a small bowl, mix baking soda, salt and cinnamon.

3. Blend the pitted dates, bananas, fresh fresh eggs, , oil and vinegar in a food processor.

4. In a small bowl transfer the mixture from the food processor to the dry ingredients mixing it thoroughly.

5. Fold in grated carrots and nuts.

6. Scoop mixture into the paper lined muffin tins.

7. Bake 30 minutes, or until done. To test, insert a toothpick at the center of the muffin, when the toothpick comes out clean, then your muffin is done!

Crunchy Zucchini

2 tbsp. bacon grease

 2 tbsp. coconut flour

4 cups zucchini

4 small fresh eggs,

Salt and pepper to taste

1. Using a peeler shred the zucchini thinly, stopping when you reach the seeds.
2. Turn zucchini to the other side and do the same procedure.
3. Dry with paper towel to remove excess water). Set aside.
4. Beat fresh fresh eggs, in a small bowl.
5. Add coconut flour into the beaten fresh fresh eggs, , and mix together.

6. Flavor the shredded zucchini with salt and pepper and combine it with the egg mixture.
7. Place a small pan over a medium- low heat.
8. When the pan is already hot, add bacon grease to coat the pan.
9. Spoon in the mixture into the pan. Depending on the size of fritters you like.
10. Fry until golden brown and crispy.

Dates Wrapped In Crispy Bacon

Ingredients

25 almonds

25 pieces toothpick

25 slices of bacon cut into half

25 pitted dates

Procedure:

1. Preheat oven to 4 6 0 F
2. With the use of a knife open up the dates
3. Stuff one almond inside each date.

4. Wrap each date with a bacon slice. Securing it with a toothpick.

5. On a shallow baking pan, put the bacons with dates and bake for 6 minutes.
6. Turnover and bake for another 6 minutes or until bacon is crispy.
7. Serve it warm or cold.

Chocolate Banana Muffin

1/2 cup coconut oil

1/2 cup coconut flour

1 baking soda

1 tsp. salt

2 cup mashed banana

4 small fresh eggs,

1 tsp. vanilla extract

4 tbsp. raw honey

1/2 cup unsweetened cocoa powder

1/2 cup semi-sweet chocolate chips

Procedure:

1. Preheat the oven to 4 6 0 F.
2. Place paper baking cups into a muffin pan.
3. Combine the mashed banana, beaten egg, vanilla extract, and coconut oil, in a mixing bowl and mix all the ingredients well.
4. Add in coconut oil, baking soda, salt and cocoa powder. Mix and fold well until all ingredients are evenly blended.
5. Spoon in the batter into each paper cup.
6. Sprinkle the chocolate chips on top.
7. Bake for 30 to 25 minutes or until done. To test if it is done, insert a toothpick in the middle of the muffin if it comes out mostly clean, then it is done!

Baked Zucchini Parmigianino

- 2 zucchinis, thinly sliced
- 2 cup of Parmigiano-Reggiano grated
- 2 teaspoon of dried oregano
- Salt and pepper

- 4 small fresh fresh eggs,
- 2 cup of almond flour
- 2 cup of ground almonds

Preparation

1. Preheat oven to 450F. Line a small baking dish with parchment paper.
2. In a small bowl combine the oregano, Parmigiano-Reggiano cheese, season with salt and pepper. Set aside.
3. Pour the almond flour in a separate bowl.
4. In another bowl, whisk the fresh fresh eggs, together.

91

5. Add salt and pepper.
6. Dip sliced zucchini in flour, then in egg mixture, then in ground almond mixture.
7. Place zucchini slices in a single layer on the baking tray. Bake 45 minutes. Serve.

Flax Meal Cinnamon Porridge

- 2 cup of water
- 2 cup of sweetener
- Ground cinnamon

- 4 Tablespoons of soft cream cheese
- 4 Tablespoons of flax meal

Preparation

1. Add listed ingredients to a microwave safe bowl. Stir well.
2. Microwave for 2 minutes. Stir again. Top with fresh berries.
3. Serve.

Feta Minty Omelette

Ingredients

- 4 ounces of feta cheese
- Salt and pepper
- Olive oil

- 4 small fresh fresh eggs,
- 6 mint leaves

Preparation

1. Preheat oven to 450F.
2. In a Little Large bowl, combine fresh fresh eggs, and feta cheese, mint leaves, salt and pepper. Whisk thoroughly.
3. In a non-stick, oven-safe frying pan, heat up some live oil. pour the egg mixture in frying pan. cook for 10 minute.
4. Remove frying pan from stove, place in oven. Cook 10 minutes.
5. Transfer omelette to a plate. Serve.

Flaxseed Savoury Waffles

- 2 cup of water
- 1 cup of melted coconut oil
- 2 Tablespoon fresh herbs

- 6 small fresh fresh eggs,
- 2 cups of ground flaxseed
- 2 Tablespoon baking powder (gluten-free)
- 1 teaspoon sea salt

Preparation

1. Pre-heat waffle maker to Little Large heat.
2. In a small bowl, combine baking powder, salt, and flaxseed. Whisk thoroughly.
3. In a seprate bowl, add fresh fresh eggs, oil and water. use handheld mixer, blend until fully comb8ined. pour egg mixture in with flaxseed mixture. stir together. let it rest 10 minutes. add the fresh herbs. stir well.
4. 1/2 cup of mixture onto waffle maker. Cook 4 – 10 minutes.
5. Serve.

Cauliflower Mozzarella Sticks

Ingredients

- 4 cups of cauliflower rice
- 2 cups + 2 cup of mozzarella cheese
- 4 small fresh fresh eggs,
- 4 cloves of minced garlic
- 4 teaspoons of fresh oregano
- Salt and pepper

Instructions

1. Preheat oven to 450F.
2. Rinse cauliflower, pat dry. Cut into florets.
3. place florets in food processor. pulse until rice-like consistency.
4. Transfer cauliflower to microwavable container. Cover and cook 25 minutes.
5. Pour cauliflower into a small bowl.

6. Add the 2 cups of mozzarella cheese, fresh fresh eggs, , oregano, salt, pepper and garlic. Stir together.
7. Line two small baking trays with parchment paper.
8. Spread mixture in single even layer on the baking trays.
9. Bake 30 minutes, until golden brown.
10. Remove trays from oven.
11. Sprinkle remaining cup of mozzarella cheese over cauliflower.
12. Return to oven for 6 minutes, until cheese melts.

Remove from oven. Let it rest for 10 minutes. Slice into sticks.

13. Side with marinara sauce. Serve.

Pistachio And Leek Muffins

Ingredients:

- 2 cup of millet flour
- 1 cup of tapioca flour
- 2 teaspoon of baking powder
- 4 Tablespoons of olive oil
- 4 cups of milk
- 2 small fresh fresh eggs,
- 2 leeks, chopped and washed
- 1 cup of chopped pistachios

Instructions

1. Preheat oven to 450F. Line muffin tin with paper liners.
2. In a small bowl, combine baking powder, flour and salt. Whisk thoroughly.

3. In a separate bowl, combine milk, fresh fresh eggs, and oil whisk thoroughly.

4. Pour egg mixture into flour mixture. Stir until combined.

5. Add half the pistachios and leeks. Stir well.

6. Fill muffin cup ¾ full. Sprinkle rest of chopped pistachios over top.

7. Bake 30 minutes, until golden brown. Cool for 30 minutes. Serve.

Flaxseed Cottage Pancakes

Ingredients

- 1 cup of ground flax seed meal
- 4 Tablespoons of cottage cheese
- 2 small fresh fresh eggs,
- 2 Tablespoons of butter
- 1 cup of heavy cream
- 1/2 teaspoon of gluten-free baking powder
- Coconut oil or olive oil for frying

Instructions

1. In a small bowl combine all the ingredients. Whisk together thoroughly
2. In a non-stick frying pan, heat the oil.
3. Spoon 3/4 cup of batter onto frying pan.

4. cook 2 minutes per side.
5. Transfer onto plate. Serve with fresh berries or (keto-friendly) syrup.

Baked Fresh Fresh Eggs, With Spinach And Mushrooms

Ingredients

- 4 cups of sliced mushrooms
- 2 coarsely chopped green bell pepper
- 2 Tablespoons of extra virgin olive oil
- Salt and pepper

- 4 small fresh fresh eggs,
- 4 cups of chopped spinach

Instructions

1. Preheat oven to 450F. Grease 8x8 baking dish with olive oil.
2. Place bell peppers, spinach, and mushrooms in baking dish.
3. **Carefully crack the fresh fresh eggs over the vegtables. Season with salt and pepper.**
4. **Bake until the whites are set, approximately 25 minutes.**
5. **Remove from oven. Transfer to plates. Serve.**

Creamy Cheese Brussel Sprouts

Ingredients

- 2 Tablespoons of extra virgin olive oil
- 2 teaspoons of organic fresh fresh lemon juice
- Salt and pepper

- 30 Brussel sprouts
- 4 cloves of garlic, minced
- ¾ cup of cream cheese

Preparation

1. Rinse Brussel sprouts in cold water. Remove stem.
2. Heat olive oil in non-stick frying pan.
3. Add minced garlic and Brussel sprouts. Saute until tender.
4. Stir in cream cheese and fresh lemon juice.

5. Transfer to bowls. Serve.

Greens And Red Hot Salad

Ingredients

- 4 Little Large beets, sliced into small wedges
- 8 cloves of garlic, minced
- 4 Tablespoons of olive oil
- 2 Tablespoon of finely chopped fresh thyme

- 4 pounds of red cabbage, sliced into small wedges
- 4 pounds of Brussel sprouts, sliced into small wedges

Instructions

1. Place chopped vegetables and garlic in pressure cooker.

2. Add the salt, pepper, thyme, and oil. Stir.
3. Set the cooker on saute. Cook for 30 minutes on high pressure.
4. Once ready, select natural release. Allow pressure to go down naturally.
5. Transfer vegetables to a platter. Serve.

Spinach Puree And Swiss Chard

Ingredients

- 4 Tablespoons of extra virgin olive oil
- 4 cups of water
- 1/2 cup of cream cheese
- Salt and pepper

- 1 pound of swiss chard
- 2 pound of baby spinach leaves
- 2 cup of cauliflower florets
- 2 leek

Instructions

1. Rinse the leek. Dice into thick slices.
2. Heat olive oil in non-stick frying pan. Add cauliflower and leek. Cook for 4 minutes.
3. Add spinach leaves, swiss chard, salt and pepper.
4. Simmer 30 minutes.

5. Allow vegetables to cool down 25 minutes.
6. Transfer to food processor. Blend into a soup. Return to the stove.
7. Stir in cream cheese and water. Heat 10 minutes.
8. Pour into bowls. Serve.

Basil Zucchini Noodles

Ingredients

- 4 cloves of garlic, mashed
- 2 teaspoon of red pepper flakes
- 1 bell red pepper, chopped
- Salt and pepper

- 4 Tablespoons of chopped fresh basil
- 2 cups of zucchini noodles
- 4 Tablespoons of extra virgin olive oil

-

Instructions

1. Use a spiralizer to turn zucchini into noodles.
2. Heat olive oil in non-stick frying pan. Add garlic, red pepper flakes, red pepper. Sauté for 2-4 minutes, until garlic releases aroma.
3. Add zucchini noodles. Stir well. Cook 4 minutes.

4. Transfer zucchini noodle mix to a plate. Garnish with basil. Serve.

Sour Braised Artichokes

Ingredients

- 2 Tablespoons of melted coconut butter
- Water
- Salt and pepper
- Fresh chopped thyme

- 4 artichokes
- 4 Tablespoons of fresh lemon juice

Instructions

1. Rinse artichokes and trim. Remove leaves until light yellow leaves are left.

Slice off top third of artichoke, trim end of the stem.

2. Place artichokes, fresh lemon juice, melted coconut butter and salt in slow cooker.
3. Cover and cook on high 2 hours, or low 4 hours, until artichokes are fork tender.
4. Transfer to platter. Garnish with chopped thyme. Serve.

Mushroom & Broccoli Mix

Ingredients

- 2 cups of thinly sliced button mushrooms
- 4 cups of broccoli
- 2 Tablespoons of minced garlic
- 1 teaspoon of dried oregano
- 4 Tablespoons of grated Parmesan
- Salt and pepper

Instructions

1. Preheat oven to 450F. Line Little Large baking dish with parchment paper.
2. In a small bowl, combine mushrooms and broccoli. Coat with olive oil.
3. Season with salt, pepper, and oregano.
4. Transfer broccoli and mushrooms to baking dish. Bake 30 minutes.
5. Serve.

Bok Choy Warm Salad

Ingredients

- 2 Tablespoons of olive oil
- 2 Tablespoons of fresh-squeezed lime juice
- Salt and pepper

- 2 bunch of trimmed bok choy
- 2 cups of water

Instructions

1. Place bok choy in pressure cooker. Add enough water to cover.
2. Close lid. Set pressure on high.
3. Cook 8 minutes.
4. Once cooked, allow pressure to drop naturally, approximately 25 minutes.
5. Transfer to serving platter. Drizzle lime juice and oil over.
6. Sprinkle salt and pepper. Serve.

Asparagus And Artichoke Salad

Ingredients

- 2 ounce of chopped pistachio nuts
- 2 small egg white
- 4 teaspoons of chopped green onions + 2 green fresh onion for garnish, chopped
- Juice from 2 fresh lemon
- Salt and white pepper

- 25 tender, fresh green asparagus (woodsy stem removed, rinsed)
- 8 fresh, Little Large artichokes
- 4 Tablespoons of extra virgin olive oil
- 2 cloves of garlic, peeled and chopped

Instructions

1. In a small pot, fill to ¾, add juice from half the fresh lemon and sprinkle of salt.

2. Peel off leaves from the artichoke. Set hearts aside. Place artichoke leaves in boiling water. Cook 410 minutes. Once boiled, rinse under cold water.

3. Place in food processor. Add rest of fresh lemon juice, half a glass of water, pinch of salt and pepper, pistachios, green onions, garlic, and egg white. Blend for 2 minute. Add olive oil slowly. Continue to blend until Little Large consistency.

4. Cut up artichoke hearts and arrange on plate. Place asparagus over top. Drizzle sauce over artichokes and asparagus. Garnish with fresh green onions. Serve.

Broiled Fresh Fresh Eggs,

Ingredients

- 4 small fresh fresh eggs,
- 6 Tablespoons of heavy cream
- 2 Tablespoon of extra virgin olive oil
- 2 Tablespoon of parmesan cheese
- 1/2 cup button mushrooms, sliced
- 1/2 cup of baby spinach
- 2 pinch of red pepper flakes
- Salt and pepper

Instructions

1. Preheat broiler to 450F. Rinse mushrooms, pat dry.
2. In a small non-stick, oven-safe frying pan, heat the oil. Fry the fresh fresh eggs, on one side for 4 minutes. Set fresh fresh eggs, aside for the moment.

3. Pour half the heavy cream in the pan. Add mushrooms. Simmer for 4 minutes.

4. Stir in rest of heavy cream. Add Parmesan cheese. Stir well.

5. Place under broiler 4 minutes.

6. Pull pan out of oven. Add spinach leaves and red pepper flakes. Stir well.

7. Return fresh fresh eggs, to the pan. Place pan under broiler 2-4 minutes.

8. Pull pan from oven. Sprinkle parmesan cheese over top.

9. Garnish with fresh spinach leaves. Serve.

Cheesy Fried Eggplant Slices

Ingredients

- 2 cup of grated Parmesan cheese
- 1 cup of coconut oil or butter
- Garlic powder
  Salt and pepper

- 2 eggplant
- 2 small egg
- 2 cup of almond flour

Instructions

1. Rinse the eggplant, pat dry. Slice in 1 inch thickness. Arrange on a plate.
2. Sprinkle with salt. Let sit for 45 minutes.
3. In a small bowl, whisk the egg. In a separate bowl, combine Parmesan

cheese, garlic powder, almond flour, salt and pepper. Stir well.

4. Heat butter or oil in a non-stick frying pan over Little Large heat.

5. Dip slice of eggplant in egg, then flour. Fry until crispy and golden brown.

6. Place cooked eggplant on a paper towel lined plate to drain excess oil.

7. Serve.

Egg with Power Greens and Sweet Potato Casserole

Ingredients

- 2 peeled sweet potatoes, diced
- 2 diced green fresh onion
- 1/2 cup of coconut milk
- 2 teaspoon of garlic powder
- 1/2 teaspoon of nutmeg
- Salt and pepper
- Seasoning of your choice

- 8 small fresh fresh eggs,
- 1 teaspoon of coconut oil
- 4 cups of power greens

Instructions

1. Preheat oven to 450F. Grease casserole dish with coconut oil.
2. In a small bowl, whisk fresh eggs, . Add onions, sweet potato, coconut milk,

power greens and seasoning. Pour egg mixture in dish.

3. Place dish in the oven. Bake 410 minutes.
4. Remove dish from the oven. Cover with foil. Bake 30 more minutes.
5. Remove from oven. Separate onto plates. Serve.

Mushrooms Roasted With Herbs & Parmesan

Ingredients

- 2 Tablespoons of mashed garlic
- 2 Tablespoon of fresh parsley
- 2 Tablespoons of fresh basil
- 2 Tablespoon of fresh thyme
- Salt and pepper

- 2 pound of Cremini mushrooms
- 2 can of diced tomatoes
- 2 cups of grated Parmesan cheese
- 2 Tablespoons of ghee

Instructions

1. Preheat the oven to 450F. Rinse the mushrooms, pat dry. Slice off stems.
2. In a small non-stick, oven-safe frying pan, melt the ghee.

3. Sauté the mushrooms for 10 minutes. Season with salt and pepper.

4. In a Little Large bowl, combine the herbs, tomatoes, salt and pepper. Stir mixture in with mushrooms. Sprinkle Parmesan cheese over top. Bake 30 minutes.

5. Remove from oven. Divide on plates. Serve.

Roasted Sweet Potatoes And Cardamom

Ingredients

- 4 chopped green onions
- Handful of shallots
- Salt and white pepper
- Olive oil

- 21 pounds of sweet potatoes
- 2 Tablespoons of softened coconut butter
- 1 teaspoon of ground cardamom

Instructions

1. Preheat the oven to 450F.
2. Heat coconut butter in small non-stick, oven-safe frying pan over Little Large heat. Sautee onions for 4 minutes.
3. Season with salt and pepper.
4. Peel the potatoes, dice into cubes. Place in a Little Large bowl.

5. Peel the shallots, add to potatoes. Add cardamom and butter.
6. Stir. Season with salt and pepper. Add ingredients to oven-safe frying pan.
7. Bake until tender, approximately 2 hour. Serve.

Fresh Lemon Green Beans & Caper Vinaigrette

Ingredients

- 2 Tablespoons of chopped capers
- Zest and juice from 2 fresh lemon
- Salt and pepper

- 2 pound of trimmed fresh green beans
- 4 Tablespoons of olive oil

Instructions

1. In a small bowl, whisk the fresh lemon juice, capers, oil, salt and pepper.
2. Boil a small pot of water, add 2 tablespoon of salt.
3. Cook the green beans until tender, approximately 4-6 minutes.
4. Drain the beans.
5. Rinse in cold water.

128

6. Drizzle caper vinaigrette over beans, toss to coat. Transfer to plates. Serve.

Garlic Scallops

Ingredients

- 1/2 cup of roughly chopped Italian parsley
- Sea salt
- Black pepper
- 1/2 teaspoon of red pepper flakes
- 2 pinch of sweet paprika
- 2 teaspoon of extra virgin olive oil

- 2 pound of small scallop
- 1/2 cup of clarified ghee butter
- 6 cloves of grated garlic
- 2 small fresh lemon
- Zest from 2 small fresh lemon

Instructions

1. Use paper towels to pat dry the scallops. Place in a Little Large bowl.
2. Coat with olive oil. Season with sweet paprika, red pepper flakes, black pepper and sea salt. Toss to coat evenly.
3. Heat a small frying pan on Little Large heat. Melt the ghee. Add the scallops. Cook 2 minutes per side, until golden brown.
4. Add garlic to frying pan. Take pan off stove. Stir ingredients for 45 seconds.
5. Squeeze half of the fresh lemon juice over scallops. Sprinkle fresh lemon zest, parsley and extra virgin olive oil over scallops. Stir.
6. Side with noodles or crusty bread. Serve.

Crustless, Feta, Mushroom Quiche

Ingredients

- 2 cup of milk
- 2 ounces of feta cheese
- 1/2 cup of grated Parmesan
- 1 cup of shredded mozzarella
- Salt & pepper

- 8 ounces of button mushrooms, thinly sliced
- 2 clove of garlic, minced
- 25 ounces of thawed frozen spinach
- 4 small fresh fresh eggs,

Instructions

1. Preheat oven to 450F. Squeeze excess water out of thawed spinach.

2. Heat some cooking oil in a small non-stick frying pan over Little Large heat.

3. Add garlic and mushrooms. Sauté until tender, approximately 8 minutes.

4. Grease a small pie dish with non-stick spray. Arrange spinach along bottom of pie dish. Pour mushrooms and garlic over spinach. Crumble feta cheese over top.

5. In a small bowl, whisk together milk, fresh fresh eggs, , and Parmesan cheese. Lightly season with pepper. Pour egg mixture on top of ingredients in pie dish.

6. Sprinkle mozzarella over the top.

7. Place pie dish on a baking tray. Place it into the oven. Bake for

approximately 46 minutes, until golden brown.

8. Remove from oven. Let it rest for 6 minutes before slicing. Serve.

Mouthwatering Paleo Chocolate Chunk Banana Bread

Ingredients:

- 1 a cup of coconut flour
- 1 a teaspoon of cinnamon
- 2 teaspoon of baking powder
- 2 teaspoon of vanilla extract
- Just a pinch of salt
- 6 ounce of chopped up dark chocolate

- 4 pieces of Banana complete mashed
- 4 pieces of fresh fresh eggs,
- 1 cup of almond butter
- 4 tablespoon of melted coconut oil

Preparation:

1. Start off by greasing up a 10 " x 6 " loaf pan and pre-heat your oven to a temperature of 4 6 0 degree Fahrenheit

2. Take a small sized bowl and toss in the mashed banana, coconut oil, fresh fresh eggs, , vanilla extract and nut butter according to the specified amounts in the ingredients and mix them nicely

3. Next add in your cinnamon, coconut flour, baking soda, seas salt and baking powder to the previously mixed wet ingredients

4. Once the batter is ready, pour that into the previously prepared pan and spread everything nicely

5. Bake for about 40 minutes if you have chosen to go for a square pan or 60 minutes if you have gone for a loaf pan

6. Check with a tooth pick and then remove it from the oven once done.

7. Allow it to cool on the wire rack for half an hour and flip out the tasty delight!

Awesome Coconut Flour Pancakes

Ingredients:

- 1/2 cup of coconut milk
- 1 teaspoon of vanilla extract
- 1/2 cup of coconut flour
- 1/2 teaspoon of tartar cream
- 1/9 teaspoon of baking soda
- 1/9 teaspoon of sea salt

- 2 teaspoon of extra virgin coconut oil
- 2 tablespoon of raw honey
- 4 pieces of small fresh fresh eggs,

Preparation:

1. The first step here is to pre-heat your oven to a temperature of 4 6 0 degree Fahrenheit

2. Take a small sized bowl and mix up all of the ingredients

3. Grease up your muffin tin using the coconut oil or better use fine paper liners if possible

4. Divide up your previous batter into 10 separate muffin tins

5. Bake for about 50 minutes until the muffin has gained a nice golden texture

6. Remove and let it cool for a while on the baking rack and eat!

Sweet Potato Paleo Muffins

Ingredients:

- 1/2 cup of chopped up dried figs
- 1 a cup of chopped up walnuts
- ¾ cup of almond flour
- 1/9 cup of maple syrup
- 2 teaspoon of cinnamon
- 1/9 teaspoon of nutmeg
- 2 teaspoon of baking powder
- 2 pieces of egg

- ¾ cup of mashed sweet potato
- 1 a cup of shredded carrot
- 1 cup of grated apple
- 1 a cup of shredded coconut
- 1 a cup of raisins

Preparation:

1. The first step here is to mix up the coconut oil and honey and cream them together. Then gently keep adding the fresh fresh eggs, one at a time
2. Then pour in the vanilla and coconut milk while mix everything until a nice smooth consistency has been achieved
3. Pour in the coconut flour then again mix it until smooth
4. Once mixed, then pour in the tartar cream, salt and baking soda
5. Mix everything gently
6. Take a ladle and finely pour small portions of your batter into a crepe pan prepared with ghee or butter and put it on Little Large heat
7. Once the bottom has a nice brown consistency, flip it up
8. Serve hot with a fine drizzle of delicious maple syrup

Crunchy Blueberry Coconut French Toast

Ingredients:

- 2 cup of fresh blueberries
- 2 cup of unsweetened shredded coconut

For the Sauce

- 2 cups of blueberries
- ¾ cup of water
- 2 teaspoon of honey
- 2 tablespoon of fresh lemon juice

- 2 pound of loaf bread
- 3 cup of coconut milk
- 6 pieces of fresh fresh eggs,
- 2 teaspoon of cinnamon
- 1 teaspoon of salt

Preparation:

1. Take a 10 x 2 4 dimension pan and grease it up nicely
2. Take your and cut them into nice 2 inch chunks and place them finely in the 10 inch by 2 4 inch pan
3. Take a separate bowl and toss in the fresh fresh eggs, , salt, milk alongside cinnamon and mix them together
4. Take the previously created mixture and pour them in to bread until they are evenly coated
5. Sprinkle some coconut and let it marinade in your fridge throughout the whole night
6. Gently pre-heat your oven to 4 6 0 degree Fahrenheit once you are ready to cook
7. Take a cup and mix in about 2 cup of blue berries to the prepared French toast and finely place it inside your oven

8. It should take about 40 minute to bake until it has a nice brown texture
9. Take a small skillet and toss in all the ingredients listed under your blueberry sauce section and boil it up
10. Gently reduce the heat to low after boiled and simmer for another 25 minutes
11. Pour in the sauce on top of your French toast and serve with blueberry sauce

Glorious Breakfast Casserole

Ingredients:

- 8 ounce of sliced up mushroom
- 25 ounce of Italian sausage
- 25 pieces of fresh fresh eggs,
- Green piece of fresh onion
- Salt as needed
- Pepper as needed

- 2 small diced up sweet potato
- 1/2 of a chopped up fresh onion
- 2 clove of crushed up garlic
- About 4 tablespoon of olive oil

Preparation:

1. Start off by taking a small sized pan and sauté your garlic and fresh onion in a good amount of olive oil until they sport a nice translucence texture

2. Toss in the deiced up sweet potatoes and cook them for 30 minutes until a nice tender texture has been achieved

3. Once done, remove the pan and toss the contents into your baking dish

4. Pour in some more oil to the pan and toss in the sliced up mushroom and sauté them until finely browned up.

5. Then season them with pepper and salt and add them to the baking dish only to create a second layer

6. Lastly, toss in your sausages and cook them finely in your pan and season with pepper and salt as well only to

toss them in you baking dish to create a final upper layer

7. Once your dish is prepared, pre-heat your oven to 4 6 0 degree Fahrenheit.

8. Take a bowl and whisk in your fresh fresh eggs, and pour them over your casserole mixture in the baking dish

9. Let the casserole bake for about 8 0 minutes until you notice that the fresh fresh eggs, are no longer running around

Sunny Tropical Sunrise Smoothie

Ingredients:

- 1 of a frozen banana
- 1 of a frozen banana
- ¾ cup of frozen strawberries
- 1 a cup of water
- a few ice cubes

- 1 a cup of fresh orange juice
- ¾ cup of frozen mango
- 1/2 cup of water

Portion 2

Preparation:

1. Notice that here the ingredients here are divided into two portions. Firstly blend up all of the ingredients listed in portion one and set it aside

2. Then take all of the ingredients of portion 2 and blend them up.

147

3. Pour half of the portion 2 mixture to the cup of portion 2 and mix them together

4. Once a orange pinkish texture has been achieved, very slowly pour the mixture into the cup with portion 2

5. Then take the portion 2 mixture and set it aside only to slowly pour it into a cup

Mouthful Of Pumpkin Smoothie

Ingredients:

- 2 dates
- 1/9 teaspoon of ground ginger
- 1/2 teaspoon of cinnamon
- Just a pinch of nutmeg

- 2 piece of ripe banana
- 1 a cup of pumpkin puree
- 2 cups of almond milk
- 2 tablespoon of peanut butter
- 6 ice cubes

Preparation:

1. Unlike the previous juice recipe, this one is not complicated at all! Just take your ingredients and toss them in a blender

2. Blend until they have gained the desired consistency and serve cold!

Crunchy Homemade Granola

Ingredients:

- 2 cup of unsweetened shredded coconut
- 2 cup of dried cranberries
- 2 egg white light beaten up
- 2 tablespoon of water
- 4 tablespoon of grapeseed oil
- 1/2 cup of honey
- 2 teaspoon of vanilla extract
- 1 a teaspoon of ground cinnamon
- 1 a teaspoon of kosher salt

- 2 cups of raw walnuts
- 2 cups of raw cashew
- 2 cup of raw pumpkin seeds

Preparation:

1. Start off by pre-heating your oven to a temperature of 4 00 degree Fahrenheit and take a baking sheet only to line it up with parchment paper

2. Toss in the first 4 ingredients listed in the list into a food processor and pulse them until they are finely chopped

3. Take a small sized mixing bowl and whisk up your egg whites

4. Pour the grape seed oil, vanilla extract, honey, cinnamon and pinches of salt to the previously created egg white mixture and whisk everything again

5. In this mixture, toss in the chopped up nut into your mixing bowl alongside the dried cranberries and the specified portion of shredded coconut

6. Mix everything to coat the nuts properly

7. Once your granola mixture if ready, spread out the mixture on a parchment-lined baking sheet and bake it for about 45 minutes until a fine golden-brown texture has been achieved

8. Once done, take it out and let it rest 25 minutes extra to make sure that a nice clustering takes place

9. Once everything is cooled up, store them and eat with yogurt or milk

Healthy Taco Salad In A Mason Jar

Ingredients:

- 2 small sized avocado
- 2 juiced up lime
- 2 cup of salsa
- 2 cup of chopped up Roma tomatoes
- 1 a cup of chopped up cucumber
- 1 a cup of roughly chopped up cilantro
- Fresh spinach
- 2 quart of wide mouth sized mason jars
- Salt as needed

- 2 tablespoon of divided up olive oil
- 8 ounce of chicken breast cut into bite sized portions
- 2 cups of small carrots sliced up
- 2 sliced up small red bell pepper
- 1   a cup of roughly chopped up fresh onion

- 2 teaspoon of minced garlic
- 2 teaspoon of cumin seed

Preparation:

1. This recipe will first require you to take a small skillet and pour in about 1 tablespoon of olive oil and heat it over Little Large

2. Toss in the chicken breast and cook them until they are nicely golden brown in texture

3. Pour in 1 tablespoon of olive oil again into another pan and heat it over Little Large high.

4. In this pan, cook the carrots for 4 minute,

5. Bring down the heat to Little Large and add in the pepper, garlic, fresh onion and cook them again until finely charred

155

6. While the vegetables are begin cooked, take your cumin seed and place it in a small sized dry pan and place it over Little Large /high heat only to toast them for 2 minutes until golden brown texture

7. Gently transfer them from there to a cutting board only to crush them nicely

8. Take the crushed seeds and toss them into the vegetable mix and season using a bit of salt and mix everything before removing the heat

9. Scoop up your avocado and a measure lime juice into the food processor and blend everything until nicely smooth

10. Then, take your mason jar and pour 1 cup of salsa in the bottom.

11. Take your avocado and lime mix and place it on top

12. Then toss the cumin, prepared vegetables and the chicken

13. Tightly pack everything and follow them with the chopped up tomatoes, cucumbers and top it off with just a bit more cilantro leave

Close it up and refrigerate before swallowing up!

Crunchy Lettuce Tacos With Chipotle Chicken

Ingredients:

- 2 teaspoon of finely chopped up chipotle
- 1 a teaspoon of cumin
- Pinch of brown sugar
- Lettuce as needed
- Fresh coriander leaves
- Sliced up pickle jalapeno chilies
- Slices of guacamole
- Fresh pieces of tomato slices
- Lime wedges

- 400g of skinless chicken breast cut into strips
- A splash of olive oil
- 2 piece of finely sliced red fresh onion
- 2 piece of 400g tomato tin

Preparation:

1. For this recipe, start off by heating up your olive oil in a non-stick frying pan and tossing in the chicken only to fry them until a fine golden brown texture has been achieved

2. Keep it aside then and toss in your tomatoes, sugar, cumin, chipotle in another pan and simmer them for about 30 minutes until a fine tomato sauce start to get thick edges

3. Into the sauce mixture, toss in your fried chicken and cook for 6 minutes

4. Assemble everything into separate plates and keep them ready for the taco making process

5. Take your taco shell and insert the ingredients according to your desire and squeeze a bit of fresh lemon to top it off.

Spicy Cuban Picadillo Lettuce Wraps

Ingredients:

- 2 teaspoon of ground cumin
- 1 a teaspoon of ground cinnamon
- 2   piece of 2 4 ounce can of whole tomatoes
- 1/2 cup of currants
- 2 tablespoon of green olive
- 2 tablespoon of drained capers
- 2 tablespoon of olive brine

- 2 pound of grass fed ground beef
- 2 tablespoon of coconut oil
- 2 .6 cup of diced up fresh onion
- 1 a teaspoon of salt
- 2   teaspoon of freshly ground black pepper

For the Pico De Gallo

- 1 a cup of minced red fresh onion
- 1/2 cup of diced tomatoes
- 2 tablespoon of minced cilantro
- 2 teaspoon of fresh lime juice
- Salt as needed

Serving

- Cooked up brown rice
- Chopped up cilantro
- Lettuce as needed

Preparation:

1. Take a small sized skillet and place it over Little Large heat only to toss in the beef and keep stirring it occasionally

2. Pour in the oil to the pan and toss further onions to cook everything until

it has been finely softened which should take no more than 4 -4 minutes

3. Add in the bell pepper and cook for another 4 minutes until nicely fragrant

4. Take another pan and toss in the cooker beef, currants, canned tomatoes, diced olives, olive brine and capers and bring the whole mix to a nice boil

5. Once boiled, reduce the heat and simmer it for about 2 0-25 minutes at low temperature

6. On the side, prepare your pico de Gallo by combining the minced up shallot, cilantro, chopped tomato and lime juice with just a pinch of salt as ending

Healthy California Turkey And Bacon Lettuce Wraps With Basil Mayo

Ingredients:

For the Pico De Gallo

- 4 slices of gluten free cooked bacon
- 2 thinly sliced avocado
- 2 thinly sliced Roma tomato

- 2 head of iceberg lettuce
- 4 slices of gluten free deli turkey

Serving

- 2 teaspoon fresh lemon juice
- 2 chopped up garlic cloves
- Salt as needed
- Pepper as needed

- 1 a cup of gluten free mayonnaise

- 6 small pieces of torn basil leaves

Preparation:

1. Take a small sized food processor to combine all of the ingredients listed under Basil Mayo and process them until very smooth

2. Take your small lettuce leaves and layer about 2 slice of turkey and slather alongside the previously prepared Basil Mayo

3. On another layer, add in a second slice of turkey and follow it thoroughly with a bacon adding a few slices of tomato and avocado

4. Season them with a some pepper and salt and fold them nicely into a burrito.

Savory Steak With Sriracha Lettuce Wraps

Ingredients:

- 2 tablespoon of sriracha
- 2 teaspoon of coconut aminos
- Sesame oil for drizzle
- Green onions for garnish
- A handful of pea shoots
- Small pieces of romaine leaves

- 2 pound of fajita strips diced up into 1 inch bites
- Small sized fresh onion diced up
- 4 diced up cloves of garlic
- 2 diced up bell pepper

Preparation:

Take a hot pan and pour in some oil and heat it for 45 seconds

Take your fajita meat and cook them on high for about 2 minutes

Add in the pepper and fresh onion and keep cooking them on high making sure to toss them occasionally for about 6 minutes until a brown texture has been achieved

Then toss in the sesame oil, garlic, sriracha, peas shoot and coconut aminos

Once the meat has finely absorbed the sauce, turn off the heat

The Best Cajun Shrimp Noodle Bowl

Ingredients:

- 1 a teaspoon of Himalayan Sea Salt
- Dash of red pepper flakes
- 2 teaspoon of garlic granules
- 2 teaspoon of fresh onion powder

- 4 cloves of crushed garlic
- 4 tablespoon of grass fed butter
- 20-25 pieces of jumbo shrimps

For the Cajun Seasoning

- 2 sliced red pepper
- 2 sliced up fresh onion
- 2 tablespoon of grass fed butter

- 2 teaspoon of paprika
- Dash of cayenne pepper
  For Others

- 2 small pieces of spiraled zucchinis

168

Preparation:

1. Start off Spiralizing your Zucchini using a fine Spiralizer

2. Take a bowl and toss in the ingredients of the Cajun seasoning and toss the shrimp as well

3. Take a pan and heat up the garlic and butter

4. Toss in the fresh onion and red pepper in that mixture and sauté for about 4 minutes

5. Toss in the Cajun shrimp and cook until nicely opaque

6. Take a separate heating pan heat up the leftover tablespoon of butter and again lightly sauté your Zucchini noodles for about 4 minutes

7. Finely place your Zucchini noodles in a bowl and top it off with your garlic Cajun shrimp and vegetable mixture.

Quick Paleo Egg Roll In A Bowl

Ingredients:

- 1/2 cup of coconut aminos
- 2 tablespoon of sesame oil
- 2 minced up garlic cloves
- 4 pieces of diced up green onions
- 2 small sized head of a cabbage chopped up into slices
- 2 small sized carrots
- 2 tablespoon of unflavored coconut oil

Preparation:

1. Melt up your coconut oil in a pan over medium-high heat range

2. Toss in the cabbage, followed by the carrots

3. Sautee them until finely softened

4. Toss in the aminos and sesame oil afterwards

5. Sautee them even more until even further tender and the sauce has been absorbed

6. Toss in the garlic and keep cooking until translucent and fragrant

7. On top them, toss the green fresh onion

8. Finally, on the side cook your chicken in olive oil/ coconut oil and shred it only to toss in with your salad and eat

Simplistic Anti Pasta Salad

Ingredients:

- 1 a cup of artichoke
- 1 a cup of olives
- 1 a cup of hot or sweet peppers
- Italian dressing as required

- 2 small sized head of chopped up romaine
- 4 ounce of strip cut prosciutto
- 4 ounce of cubed up salami

Preparation:

1. This is a very simple recipe which only requires you to mix up everything that has been listed throughout and toss them up the Italian dressing

Soft Skillet Chicken Thigh With Butternut Squash

Ingredients:

- Extra Virgin olive oil/ Coconut for frying
- Freshly chopped up sage
- Salt as needed
- Pepper as needed

- 1 a pound of Nitrate free bacon
- 6 boneless and skinless chicken thigh
- 2-4 cup of butternut squash cubed up

Preparation:

1. The first step here is to pre-heat your oven to about 430 degree Fahrenheit

2. Take a small sized skillet and over Little Large high heat, fry up your bacon until it is crispy

3. Take your bacon and place it on the side and crumble it when cooled

4. In the very same skillet, sauté your cubed up butternut squash in bacon grease until tender

5. Season it with pepper and salt

6. Once the squash is softened ,remove it from your skillet and place it on a nice plate

7. Add in your coconut oil to the skillet and if the level of bacon grease is low

8. Toss in the chicken thigh and cook for 25 minutes

9. Season with pepper and salt

10. Flip them over and add your squash

11. Remove the skillet from your stove and place it in your pre-heated oven

12. Bake for about 2 2-30 minutes

13. Remove and top with crumbled bacon and sage before serving hot

Sweet Paleo Turkey Potato Casserole With Eggplant And Tomato

Ingredients:

- 2 can of 8 ounce tomato paste
- 1 a teaspoon of salt
- 1 teaspoon of pepper
- 1/2 teaspoon of chili powder
- 1/2 teaspoon of cumin

- 2 and a 1 tablespoon of extra virgin olive oil
- 2 cup of unsweet almond milk
- 2 tablespoon of almond flour
- 2 tablespoon of coconut flour

- 1/9 teaspoon of oregano
- 1/9 teaspoon of ground cardamom
- 2 pound of extra lean ground turkey
- 2 Little Large sized sweet potato, peeled up and spiralized
- 2 Little Large sized eggplant sliced into 1 inch pieces
- 2 /4 cup of chopped up fresh onion
- 2 tablespoon of minced up garlic
- 2 piece of 30 ounce can of petite diced tomatoes
- 1 a teaspoon of tarragon flakes

For the Sauce

Preparation:

1. Pre-heat your oven to a temperature of 50 0degree Fahrenheit

2. Take a 8x8 inch square casserole dish and spray it with non-stick cooking spray

3. Heat up your small pan over Little Large level heat and toss in the turkey, fresh onion and garlic and cook them until finely browed making sure to break apart the turkey with a spatula

4. Stir in your tomato paste and tomatoes to the turkey mixture and add in the sweet potatoes and cook until tender

5. Take you chopped up eggplant in a bowl and toss everything with the seasonings to congregate

6. Finely place the processed eggplant on the bottom part of your casserole dish and top follow it with turkey and sweet potato mix

7. Place it inside the oven and let it bake for about 30 minutes

8. While it is being baked, heat up a small pot and bring it to boil and toss the almond, alongside olive oil and coconut flour

9. Stir in for about 2 minutes until mixture thickens and reduce your heat to Little Large high

10. Slowly add the almond milk to the pan while whisking as you stir the mixture

11. Continue whisking for the next 25 minutes until the sauce is reduced to half of its former self

12. Place your casserole back in the oven and cook for about 46 minutes until the top if browned in texture

13. Gently remove everything from the oven and top it up with even more tarragon

14. Slice the mixture in 6 pieces and serve hot

Superbly Delicious Paleo Pizza Soup

Ingredients:

- 2 diced up small fresh onion
- 35 ounce of sliced mushroom
- 2 can of 4 ounce sliced up black olives
- 2 tablespoon of dried oregano
- 2 teaspoon of garlic powder
- 1 a teaspoon of salt

- 25 ounce of sliced up chicken sausage
- 4 ounce of uncured pepperoni
- 2 can of 30 ounce marinara
- 2   can of 2 4.6   ounce fire roasted tomatoes

Preparation:

1. Take small sized saucepan and toss in the peperoni, sausage, marinara, onions, tomatoes, mushroom, oregano, olives, salt and garlic powder

2. Cook the mixture for 45 minutes over Little Large level heat and soften the mushroom and onions

Spicy Pumpkin Paleo Chili

Ingredients:

- 2 tablespoon of honey
- 4 teaspoon of chili spice
- 2 teaspoon of ground cinnamon
- 2 teaspoon of sea salt
- 4 cups of chopped up yellow fresh onion

- 8 cloves of chopped up garlic
- 2 pound of ground turkey
- 2 can of 30 ounce fire roasted tomato
- 2 cups of pumpkin puree
- 2 cup of chicken broth

Preparation:

1. Take a small sized pot and Sautee your fresh onion and garlic in poured down coconut oil for about 6 minutes

2. Toss in the ground turkey and break it up using your spatula then cook for another 6 minutes

3. Toss in the rest of the ingredients listed and bring it to simmer after mixing

4. Simmer for about 30 minutes without a lid

5. Pour in the chicken broth.

Tangy Creamy Basil And Tomato Chicken

Ingredients:

- 2 tablespoon of nutritional yeast
- 2 package of basil
- 2 tablespoon of avocado oil
- Salt as needed
- Pepper as needed
- 1 a cup of coconut milk
- 1 a teaspoon of arrowroot powder
- 1/2 cup of cold water
- 2 cup of sliced up cherry tomatoes

- 2 pound of boneless and skinless chicken breast
- 1 a yellow fresh onion
- 2 teaspoon of coconut oil

- 4 cloves of garlic
- 2 tablespoon of sunflower seeds

Preparation:

1. Heat up your coconut oil over a small sized skillet at Little Large high het and sizzle it

2. Slice up your fresh onion into fine strips and toss them in the heating pan to cook it translucent

3. Once fully translucent, toss in the chicken to your pan and cook for 25 minutes and flip the chicken only to cook for another 2 4 minutes

4. In the meantime, take a plate and toss in the garlic in a food processor bowl to finely mince it using the processor

5. Toss in the sunflower seed and pulse it yet again

6. Toss in the nutrition yeast, some salt and just a dash of pepper

7. Pulse until fully minced

8. Take a small bowl and whisk up your arrowroot powder in a water

9. Pour in the coconut milk and whist the pest mixture previously made in

10. Pour in the sauce into the chicken skillet and bring it to a fine simmer

11. Add in the sliced cherry tomatoes and allow them to simmer for a while longer, like 2-4 minutes then serve hot

CPSIA information can be obtained
at www.ICGtesting.com
Printed in the USA
BVHW090821111220
595366BV00014B/1429

9 781990 061912